FOUR HEALTH GUARDIANS

The major antioxidant nutrients—vitamins A, C and E and the trace mineral selenium—act as a quadruple-threat defense against many of the diseases we dread most, and even have been shown to avert some of the "inevitable" effects of aging. This Good Health Guide details the fascinating research behind these discoveries, the remarkable clinical results they have led to, the varied ways in which antioxidants work in the body, and, most important, how you can use them to maintain and enhance your most important possession, your health.

ABOUT THE AUTHOR AND EDITORS

Richard A. Passwater, Ph.D., with Earl Mindell, is series editor of the Good Health Guide series. He is one of the most called-upon authorities for information relating to preventive health care. A noted biochemist, he is credited with popularizing the term "supernutrition," largely as a result of having written two bestsellers on the subject—*Supernutrition: Megavitamin Revolution* and *Supernutrition for Healthy Hearts*. His other books include *Easy No-Flab Diet, Cancer and Its Nutritional Therapies, Selenium as Food & Medicine, Trace Elements, Hair Analysis and Nutrition* (with Elmer M. Cranton, M.D.) and The Good Health Guide *The Antioxidants*.

Earl Mindell, R.Ph., Ph.D. combines the expertise and working experience of a pharmacist with extensive knowledge in most of the nutrition areas. *Earl Mindell's Vitamin Bible* is now a million-copy bestseller, and his more recent *Vitamin Bible for Your Kids* may very well duplicate his first *Bible*'s publishing history. His latest book is *Shaping Up With Vitamins*. Dr. Mindell's popular *Quick & Easy Guide to Better Health* is published by Keats Publishing, as is *The Vitamin Robbers*, a Good Health Guide.

The Antioxidants

The nutrients that guard your body

Richard A. Passwater, Ph.D.

Keats Publishing, Inc. 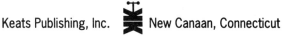 New Canaan, Connecticut

The Antioxidants is not intended as medical advice. Its intention is solely informational and educational. Please consult a medical or health professional should the need for one be indicated.

THE ANTIOXIDANTS

ISBN: 0-87983-404-8

Printed in the United States of America

Good Health Guides are published by
Keats Publishing, Inc.
27 Pine Street (Box 876)
New Canaan, Connecticut 06840

Contents

Studies over the last twenty years have shown that a group of nutrients called antioxidants can protect against cancer, heart disease, arthritis, cataracts and allergies, and at the same time slow the aging process. Some of the most important of these nutrients are vitamins A, C and E, and the trace mineral selenium.

We are still learning ways in which these common nutrients protect us from, control or even help us overcome an increasing number of seemingly totally unrelated diseases, and we are beginning to understand the common factors linking them. They are not caused by germs—bacteria or viruses—but by deleterious biochemical reactions with molecular fragments called free radicals. The process that causes these diseases, often considered to be a normal part of the aging process, is called free-radical pathology. The antioxidant nutrients block the deleterious free-radical reactions and thus protect the body.

Antioxidants are compounds that sacrifice themselves to oxygen, thus preventing it from reacting with other compounds. Antioxidant compounds have chemistries that allow them to react readily with oxygen. This ease of reaction enables antioxidant compounds to interact with free-radical generators and quench free-radical production.

The antioxidants do more than protect; they also stimulate the immune response to help fight already existing disease, and they normalize the balance of hormone-like chemicals in the body that control pain, inflammation and fever.

If you did not understand that an antibiotic such as penicillin cured a great number of diseases by destroying the bacteria that cause those diseases, you would find it difficult to believe that one drug could work against so many diseases; it's much the same with antioxidants. So let's take a brief look at the common free radical-initiated diseases, cancer, heart disease, aging, arthritis and cataracts, and then take up the role of the antioxidant nutrients in preventing or controlling those diseases.

FREE RADICALS

A free radical is an incomplete molecule, highly reactive because its electron arrangement is out of "spin" balance. Atoms, molecules and ions are more stable entities because they have more balanced electron arrangements.

The highly reactive free radicals do more damage than does a one molecule-to-one molecule reaction. Each free radical is capable of destroying an enzyme or protein molecule or even an entire cell. The damage is actually much more extensive than that because each free radical usually generates a chain of free-radical reactions, resulting in thousands of free radicals being released to destroy body components. This process is called biological magnification.

Dr. William Pryor of Louisiana State University points out several ways in which free radicals do extensive damage to our bodies. "This biological magnification occurs for two reasons. The first, and most important, is the enormous sensitivity of the cell to modifications in its heredity apparatus such as its DNA. The chromosomes, which control the reproduction of the cell, are extremely radiation-sensitive; the cytoplasm is much less so. Largely because of the sensitivity of DNA, radiation that destroys only one molecule in one million or ten million in the cell can be lethal.

"The second cause of biological magnification is that any polymeric system [one involving large numbers of similar molecules joined together] is sensitive to small chemical changes, and many important biomolecules are polymers."

Free-radical reactions leading to cell membrane damage can cause cancer, heart disease or accelerated aging.

These are five basic types of damage caused by free radicals:

1. Lipid peroxidation, in which free radicals initiate damage to fat compounds in the body, causing them to turn rancid and release more free radicals.

2. Cross-linking, in which free-radical reactions cause proteins and/or DNA molecules to fuse together.

3. Membrane damage, in which free-radical reactions destroy the integrity of the cell membrane, which in turn interferes with the cell's ability to take in nutrients and expel wastes.

4. Lysosome damage, in which free-radical reactions rupture

lysosome (cell digestive particle) membranes; these then spill into the cell and digest critical cell compounds.

5. Accumulation of the age pigment (lipofuscin), which may interfere with cell chemistry.

The most damaging agents of free-radical reactions include the superoxide, hydroxyl and lipid peroxide radicals and hydrogen peroxide.

The body defends itself against these agents with vitamin E (a general antiradical), superoxide dismutase (an enzyme that destroys the superoxide radical), catalase (an enzyme that converts hydrogen peroxide to water), and glutathione peroxidase (a selenium-containing enzyme that deactivates lipid peroxides). Each molecule of glutathione peroxidase contains four atoms of selenium. Thus selenium is a key component of the body's defense against free radicals.

CANCER

It seems that nearly every week we read that scientists have found that yet another widely encountered chemical causes cancer. But there is some good news. A moderate lifestyle and good nutrition are protective against cancer, and it's *not* true that everything causes cancer. In fact, many of the cancer-causing chemicals that we read of aren't worth worrying about. Normally, you won't eat, drink or breathe in enough of them to cause cancer. Yet if you are malnourished, your chances of getting all types of cancer increase.

Some more good news is that several vitamins and minerals have special protective properties.

• **Vitamin A and beta-carotene**, shown for forty years to be effective in treating and preventing cancers of the lung, breast, and skin.

• **Vitamin C**, estimated by one researcher to have the potential of cutting the cancer death rate by 75 percent.

• **Vitamin E** combats cancer-causing pollution and works with anti-cancer drugs.

• **Selenium**, the missing mineral—where it is absent, cancer rates soar.

A healthy body can overcome cancer, just as it can ward off cancer. Those who disagree with this statement don't fully understand what a *healthy* body is. As our understanding of nutrition and health has advanced beyond the obvious relationship of vitamin C to scurvy or vitamin B1 and beriberi, there have been many experiments that demonstrate the role of vitamins and minerals in protecting the cells against the agents that cause cancer and in stimulating the immune response to destroy cancers.

Nutritional therapy, which brings the body to its peak of immune response, in no way conflicts with surgery, radiation or chemotherapy.

Cancer is often described as a disease of civilization, but it will strike only when the body's defenses are down or when the cancer-causing agent is abnormally strong and its presence prolonged. Our strategy should be to keep our defenses up and to prevent unnecessary exposure to cancer-causing agents.

We can accomplish this by following a few simple guidelines, and by using common sense and avoiding extremes or fanaticism. The Bible summarized this wisdom thus: "Let your moderation be known unto all men" (Philippians 4:5).

Many scientists believe that cancer occurs only when the body's immune system fails. There is evidence that cells regularly grow wildly, but are detected and destroyed by the immune system.

Defective cells can grow uncontrollably. As long as nutrients are available, these cells will continue to grow and divide irregularly. Normally, antibodies are summoned which surround and isolate the premalignant cells and, with the help of macrophages (large scavenger cells), destroy them. If the body does not detect the premalignant cells as foreign, or cannot produce adequate antibodies, or if the antibodies are blocked before they do their job, then the cells develop their own blood supply and become malignant tissue.

THE IMMUNE SYSTEM AND VITAMIN A

The stimulation of the immune system is receiving increasing interest as a cure for cancer. The immune system is a complicated and poorly understood defense mechanism. It can destroy cancer unless it is weakened by poor nutrition, emotional strain or "blocking factors" formed in advanced cancers.

Researchers first noticed in 1925 that there was a relationship between a deficiency in vitamin A and cancer. Several experiments from the 1930s through the 1950s confirmed this relationship, and since then we have learned that cancer-causing chemicals can react strongly with DNA in vitamin A-deficient cells, that cancers are hard to transplant into animals adequately nourished with vitamin A, and that vitamin A is therapeutic in dealing with precancerous cells.

Scientific optimism about the effectiveness of vitamin A increased in 1974. At that time Dr. Frank Chytill of Vanderbilt University remarked, "Recent dramatic findings about vitamin A and its effects on cancer have opened up a whole new approach to cancer therapy. With vitamin A therapy, doctors may some day have a way to restore body cells to normal—rather than destroy them with surgery, chemotherapy or radiation. We now have laboratory evidence that, under certain laboratory conditions, cancers such as breast, lung, and skin tumors can be cured by treatment with vitamin A. . . . People can certainly cut their chances of getting cancer by making sure they are not deficient in vitamin A."

Dr. David Ong, a co-researcher of Dr. Chytill's at Vanderbilt, says "We know that lack of vitamin A retards normal growth, weakens the mucous linings of the body and causes night blindness. But when the proper level of vitamin A is restored, the body returns to normal. Preliminary evidence from Europe strongly indicates that vitamin A works the same way with cancer."

Dr. George Plotkin of the Massachusetts Institute of Technology adds, "A deficiency of vitamin A prevents a mucous coating from forming on the trachea, lungs, rectum, digestive system and on the inside of the skin. The vitamin A deficiency doesn't cause cancer, but it makes these areas less able to resist cancer."

Dr. Plotkin and his colleague Dr. Paul Newberne reported that giving rats ten times their usual vitamin A intake dramatically slashed their susceptibility to lung cancer.

In one of Dr. Umberto Saffioti's experiments when he was at the Chicago Medical School (he later joined the National Cancer Institute), 113 hamsters were dosed with the cigarette smoke carcinogen benzopyrene. In the 53 control animals not given extra vitamin A protection, 16 developed lung cancer. However, in the 60 vitamin A-treated animals, only one developed lung cancer and four developed benign tumors. Dr. Saffiotti had similar results with carcinogens that cause cancer in the stomach, gastrointestinal tract and uterine cervix.

Dr. E. Bjelke of the Cancer Registry of Norway found that 74 percent of the men with lung cancer were in the lowest third of the population, ranked by vitamin A intake. He also found that vitamin A especially helped smokers living in cities. Vitamin A-deficient city dwellers have three times the lung cancer rate of better-nourished city dwellers.

In a December 1977 interview Dr. Sporn discussed with me

the effects of vitamin A deficiency and his tests of more efficient vitamin A derivatives. "If you are vitamin A-deficient, there is no question that you may be more susceptible to development of cancer, but you do not need to take a lot of vitamin A to correct a deficiency. Any sort of multivitamin tablet will alleviate a deficiency state. That includes keeping your mucous membranes and respiratory tract in proper working order.

"I am not recommending that anybody take megadoses of vitamin A, but probably one of the best investments you can make in your food budget is to spend a few cents a day for that multivitamin capsule."

Dr. Sporn pointed out, "Well over half of all human cancer starts in epithelial tissue, the tissue that forms the lining of organs, forms glands such as mammary glands, skin, and passages in the body. The respiratory tract, the digestive tract, the urinary tract and the reproductive tract are all lined with epithelial tissue. And all of the specialized cells that form epithelial tissue depend on vitamin A for their normal development.

"But as far as vitamin A deficiency is concerned, there is work way back in the 1920s by D. S. B. Wolbach of Harvard which suggests a relationship between vitamin A deficiency and cancer. Dr. Wolbach pointed out that there were similarities between the cancerous process and what goes on in tissues that are vitamin A-deficient in terms of loss of control in cell differentiation. The problem that exists in cancer was pointed out over fifty years ago."

There is a debate over how vitamin A and its derivatives control early precancerous stages to prevent the development of cancer.

I asked Dr. Sporn if the retinoids (vitamin A and similar compounds) destroy a precancerous cell or just keep it from spreading.

Dr. Sporn's answer not only sheds light on how vitamin A works, but strengthens the contention that cancer can be prevented or slowed with vitamins.

"We don't have all the answers to that question, so a lot of research is being done in that area now. None of the retinoids, if used appropriately, are cytotoxic [cell-killing] agents. You can kill a cell or a person with too much of anything—even salt or water. But one does not think of salt and water as toxic agents. Similarly, if used in sensible amounts, the retinoids are not toxic agents.

"They are hormone-like controllers of cell differentiation. The approach that we are trying to develop is to use them not to kill cancer cells but to control the differentiation of precancerous cells."

What Dr. Sporn means by cell differentiation is that the cells stay in a mature differentiated state, rather than reverting to the undifferentiated condition that is characteristic of cancer.

Dr. Sporn further explained, "Now whether this actually arrests the process of development of cancer or whether this causes the precancerous cells to disappear from tissue is a topic of current research.

"If all that you do is just slow down this process of development of cancer so that instead of the typical twenty-year latent period from the time people may be first exposed to a carcinogen and the time that they develop cancer, you double that latent period, then there would be twenty additional years of good life that you would be offering people.

"Now in terms of modern surgery and chemotherapy, if they get an additional five years of survival, this is considered a very major achievement. So what we are really trying to do is to slow down or prevent the development of malignancy.

"If you slow it down enough, then for practical purposes it never occurs, although the basic process of development of cancer may still be going on, but at a very, very slow rate—such that it really never causes anyone any problems.

"The latent period is like a fire that is smoldering beneath the surface. It gives no symptoms; but, if one goes and looks for precancerous [premalignant] cells, you can find evidence of the chronic disease process. The object of the preventive approach as I see it is to do something about the disease process when it is in this early smoldering stage, before you have the fire. Once you have invasive cancer, then you can't do prevention any more. You have to change your approach.

"It's pretty clear that retinoids have a hormone-like action in controlling cell differentiation. Cancer would appear to be a disease in which the gene material, DNA, has been damaged by chemicals or radiation. Usually the damage will kill the cells, but sometimes the damage leads to cancer.

"Once DNA is damaged, cancer doesn't occur immediately. It can be twenty years after DNA damage occurs before malignancy develops.

"The word retinoid is just a generic word which describes a family of substances. Within this family there are hundreds of different individual compounds. Some of the individual compounds are the naturally-occurring forms of vitamin A such as those we eat in our diet or take in vitamin pills.

"These natural forms of vitamin A are largely stored in the liver and if taken in excess, they can cause very severe liver damage and also cause other undesirable toxic side effects. There have been cases of people who have symptoms resembling brain tumor due to excessive dosages of vitamin A. Some people believe that if some is good, then some more is better.

With massive amounts of vitamin A, they can get themselves into rather severe side effects.

"Also," Dr. Sporn points out, "vitamin A does not get into all the body parts in high enough concentrations that we want for effectiveness. If you were worried about the development of bladder cancer and took a large amount of vitamin A, this would be mostly stored in the liver and would not be getting additional vitamin A to your bladder."

BETA-CAROTENE

Dr. Sporn's most recent interest has been in the natural nutrient that the body converts into vitamin A and other retinoids. This nutrient is beta-carotene, which is found in carrots and other yellow vegetables, and dark green leafy vegetables. All those vegetables said to contain vitamin A actually have not vitamin A but its precursor, beta-carotene.

The body can split a molecule of beta-carotene in half to form two molecules of vitamin A. But beta-carotene is more than just the precursor of vitamin A. Beta-carotene has its own chemistry independent of its vitamin A chemistry. Thus beta-carotene can give you all the protection of vitamin A and then some. Scientists have found that beta-carotene becomes a unique antioxidant under certain low-pressure conditions in the cell, and it is a quencher of the deleterious form of oxygen called singlet oxygen.

In February 1981 the doctor whose research first linked smoking to lung cancer reported that a diet heavy in carrots reduces the risk of lung cancer. Dr. Richard Doll, president of the British Association for Cancer Research, found that beta-carotene reduced cancer incidence in laboratory animals by forty percent.

In April 1981 Dr. Eli Seifter of the Albert Einstein College of Medicine reported research with mice showing that beta-carotene could limit or prevent growth of cancer cells. Dr. Seifter found that from two to five times as many mice not given beta-carotene developed cancer when inoculated with breast cancer cells as did the beta-carotene fed cells. When the mice were given radiation therapy plus beta-carotene, the tumors regressed completely.

SELENIUM

The trace mineral selenium may be an even more powerful protector against cancer. Hundreds of animal tests plus several epidemiological studies provide evidence of selenium's effectiveness and safety. Only a few will be cited here, but many more can be found in my book on the subject, *Selenium as Food and Medicine* (Keats Publishing, 1980).

Dr. Gerhard Schrauzer of the University of California at San Diego found that dietary selenium reduced the incidence of cancer in a strain of mice that normally have an 80–85 percent incidence of breast cancer due to a virus that they ingest with their mother's milk to only 10 percent. The eightfold-reduced incidence of cancer in Dr. Schrauzer's study is striking, but it is important to note as well that even among the 10 percent of the selenium-supplemented mice that did develop cancer, the disease did not appear until 50 percent later than among the control animals, the tumors were less malignant and the control animals' survival time was 50 percent longer. In a less cancer-prone strain of mice, the breast cancer might have been totally prevented. Many studies have led to a growing conviction of the importance of selenium in preventing and controlling cancer.

Dr. Schrauzer firmly states: "We now think that if a breast cancer patient has especially low selenium blood levels, her tendency to develop metastases is increased, her possibility for survival is diminished, and her outlook in general is poorer than if she has normal levels. The key to cancer prevention lies in assuring the adequate intake of selenium, as well as of other essential trace elements."

In 1969, Dr. Raymond Shamberger of the Cleveland Clinic and Dr. Doug Frost of Battleboro, Vermont, noticed an inverse relationship between the incidence of cancer and the amount of selenium in patients' blood samples. Also, the lower the level of selenium in locally grown crops, the higher the incidence of cancer.

Let's look at some of the epidemiological data. Rapid City, South Dakota, has the lowest cancer rate of any city in the United States, according to one survey. The citizens of Rapid City also have the highest measured blood selenium levels in the nation. But in Lima, Ohio, which has twice the cancer rate of Rapid City, the citizens have only 60 percent of the blood selenium levels of those in Rapid City.

In another study, Drs. Shamberger and Willis found healthy persons between the ages of 50 and 71 to average 21.7 micrograms of selenium per 100 milliliters of blood, whereas cancer patients of the same age range averaged only 16.2 micrograms per 100 milliliters. The worst cancer cases had the lowest selenium levels, 13.7, 13.9 and 14.3.

The association between high selenium levels in the diet and a lower-than-average cancer rate was suggested in a paper delivered by Dr. Christine S. Wilson, a nutritionist at the University of California, San Francisco. She told the FASEB meeting that high selenium levels in the diet may explain why the breast cancer rate is substantially lower in Asian women than in women from Western countries.

After comparing the nutrient content of an average non-Western diet supplying 2500 calories to that of a typical American diet providing the same number of calories, Wilson determined that the Western diets contained about a fourth of the selenium of the Asian diets. She says that it is also significant that the Asian diets contained much less "easily oxidizable" polyunsaturated fats (7.5 to 8.7 grams a day) than the Western diets (10 to 30 grams).

Dr. Wilson hypothesizes that it is the dietary combination of high selenium and low polyunsaturated fatty acids that may be protecting the Asian women against breast cancer. She notes that selenium is a component of the glutathione peroxidase system. Because the enzyme acts to inhibit the oxidation of unsaturated fats, it blocks the formation of peroxides and free radicals, both of which are believed to trigger various forms of cancer. The connection between a low cancer rate and high-selenium diet was reinforced by Shamberger, who says that another Cleveland Clinic survey suggests that high selenium levels appear to be associated with a corresponding decrease in deaths from cancer of the colon.

In Venezuela, the death rate from cancer of the large intestine is 3.06 per 100,000 while in the United States it is 13.69 per 100,000. Venezuela has a high selenium content in its soils, while we are low. Japan, another high-selenium country, has less breast cancer, as already mentioned, and also has a lower lung cancer death rate—12.65 per 100,000 compared to our 36.86 per 100,000.

There is even stronger evidence that selenium protects against cancer. So far, we have learned that extra selenium has reduced spontaneous cancer in mice and that epidemiological studies associate low selenium levels with high incidence of cancer.

Dr. Shamberger has also shown that painting selenium on the skin of mice near areas that had been painted with the carcinogen DMBA reduced the number of tumors normally obtained with DMBA. The selenium was neither mixed with nor painted on the same spot as the DMBA.

In one series of such nondietary experiments, the incidence of tumors dropped by 43 percent with the nonselenium-treated mice to 17 percent with the selenium-treated mice. A second part of the experiment involved different timing of the selenium application, and the incidence dropped from 89 percent in the controls to 45 percent among the selenium-treated.

In still another nondietary series, this time using the carcinogen MCA instead of DMBA, the incidence dropped from 87 percent in the controls to 68 percent in the selenium-treated mice.

In another series of experiments, the selenium was added in the diet rather than being painted on the skin. This approximates the human experience of environmental exposure to carcinogens being contained by dietary supplementation more nearly than do the painted tests.

Dr. Shamberger tested several timing schedules for beginning the diet supplementation after painting the carcinogen on the skin of the mice. The two-week delay experiment described typical results.

In one experiment testing a selenium-fortified diet against the effects of DMBA-croton oil, 14 of 35 mice on the selenium-fortified diet had tumors after twenty weeks, compared to 26 of 36 mice on the selenium-deficient diet. Those mice on the selenium-fortified diet that did get tumors took longer to develop them.

A similar experiment with the carcinogen benzopyrene showed 31 of 36 mice on a selenium-deficient diet developing cancer, opposed to only 16 of 36 mice on the selenium-fortified diet.

To more nearly simulate the ingesting of carcinogens in food or water, carcinogens can be added to the diet, and comparisons made between normal diets and selenium-fortified diets. This has been done by Drs. C. G. Clayton and C. A. Baumann with azo dyes, by Dr. J. R. Harr et al. with FAA (1972), and by myself with DMBA (1969-1972). Dr. Lee Wattenberg has done similar experiments with other antioxidants besides selenium.

My experiments were conducted with several antioxidants used in synergistic combination to provide animal protection at the lowest total dosage of antioxidants possible. The incidence of stomach cancer to be expected in mice given DMBA is 85 to 90 percent. That can be reduced to 5 to 15 percent with mixtures of water- and fat-soluble natural and synthetic antioxidants, including selenium.

In my experiments, the mice were all given the same dose of the carcinogen continually in their diets. Subgroups of the animals were then fed one of three different amounts of antioxidants as a percentage of their total diet throughout their lifespans.

Dr. Harr's group fed the animals the FAA continually as a part of their diet, during the entire experiment. Various amounts of selenium were also added to the diet and were thus fed concomitantly with the carcinogen.

They used groups of 20 mice. Group one received 150 parts per million FAA and 2.5 ppm added selenium; group two received 150 ppm FAA and 0.5 ppm added selenium; groups three received 150 ppm FAA and 0.1 ppm added selenium; and group four received 150 ppm FFA and no added selenium.

After 210 days, 80 percent of groups three and four had cancer, compared to 10 percent of group two and three percent of group one. The selenium had a definite protective effect.

At a February 1978 conference on preventing cancer, held at the National Cancer Institute in Bethesda, Maryland, considerable emphasis was given to the role of selenium in preventing cancer. In addition to the updates on the research conducted by Drs. Shamberger and Schrauzer, Dr. A. Clark Griffin, of the M.D. Anderson Hospital and Tumor Institute in Houston, reported that selenium added to drinking water, or selenium fed in the form of high-selenium yeast, can protect rats exposed to three different kinds of cancer-causing chemicals from colon and liver cancer. Dr. Griffin's group has also shown that selenium can prevent the conversion of potentially cancer-causing chemicals into other harmful forms. Experiments by Dr. Charles R. Shaw, also of M.D. Anderson Hospital, show that selenium cuts the bowel cancer rate from 87 percent down to 40 percent in animals fed carcinogens.

Many different types of laboratory experiments have been conducted and they all show that selenium is protective against cancer. Tumor cells injected into animals grow when the animals are selenium-deficient, but do not survive in selenium-fortified animals; these animals are protected against both carcinogen-induced cancer and virus-induced cancer. The research has been examined by many scientists and is considered meaningful.

VITAMIN E

Vitamin E has been shown to help prevent cancers caused by many chemicals in our environment. This is important because scientists estimate that 80 to 95 percent of human cancers are caused by environmental carcinogens.

Vitamin E also appears to lessen the harmful effects of the widely used anti-cancer drug Adriamycin. The drug has had limited usage because of its harmful side effects, but now, in combination with vitamin E, more effective dosages can safely be given to more people.

Additional vitamin E is also required by those who over-consume polyunsaturated oils on many low-cholesterol diets. These oils have been shown to be cofactors in potentiating the effect of other cancer-causing chemicals.

Vitamin E gives us a second chance by stimulating our immune response, which can destroy precancerous cells before they turn into a malignancy.

VITAMIN C

Vitamin C has several modes of action useful for preventing or controlling cancer. It strengthens the body's defenses against cancer by increasing the effectiveness of the immune system that destroys cancer cells, and makes it more difficult for cancer cells to reproduce and spread by strengthening an intercellular material called "ground substance." Vitamin C also protects us by preventing the formation of cancer-causing chemicals called nitrosamines from nitrites, and directly detoxifies still other carcinogens. Vitamin C also stimulates the production of interferon.

Not many people are familiar with the clinical evidence that has caused Dr. Linus Pauling, two-time Nobel laureate, to conclude that "a high intake of vitamin C is beneficial to all patients with cancer."

Drs. Pauling and Ewan Cameron jointly published a report on the beneficial effects of vitamin C on terminal cancer patients in 1976 in the *Proceedings of the National Academy of Science*.

The Cameron-Pauling study compared 100 terminally ill patients given 10 grams (10,000 milligrams) of vitamin C per day to 1000 other such patients. Both groups were treated identically in all ways—by the same physicians in the same hospital—except one was not given the vitamin C.

At the time the study report was prepared, those patients given vitamin C had lived more than four times longer than the matched "control" patients. The patient survival rate continued to improve long after the report was published.

Sixteen of the 100 in the vitamin C group lived more than a year as opposed to only three of the 1000 patients not given vitamin C.

These patients, now apparently healthy, were once considered terminal. The progress of their disease was such that in the considered opinion of at least two independent physicians, the continuance of any conventional form of treatment would offer no further benefit.

At the time of the 1976 report, 13 vitamin C-treated colon cancer patients had lived more than seven times as long as the 130 matched control patients, with improved quality of life and lessened pain.

The 1976 report also indicated that the vitamin C-treated breast cancer patients lived six times longer than their matched control group, and vitamin C-treated kidney cancer patients lived five times longer.

Drs. Cameron and Pauling also noted that survival time was increased by a factor of at least 20 for some 10 percent of the patients. This caused them to wonder what the results would be if treatment were started earlier and if larger amounts of vitamin C were used.

In 1983, the Mayo Clinic ran a similar test on cancer patients who had had chemotherapy and reported no benefit from the use of vitamin C. Dr. Pauling has since explained to them that vitamin C could not work in those cases because the drugs had destroyed the patients' immune systems. Mayo has now agreed to repeat the test, using patients not given the drugs.

When asked how many lives could be saved with the use of vitamin C in cancer treatment, Dr. Pauling replied, "In 1971 when I first suggested that vitamin C might be of use against cancer, I estimated that it might save 10 percent of the people who die of cancer. The reason that I was saying that was, although there are some very good arguments why vitamin C might be effective, there was very little direct evidence. There was only some epidemiological evidence at that point. Now 10 percent is 36,000 Americans a year, kept from dying of cancer. That's about a hundred a day. Today I'm around to saying that with proper use of vitamin C for cancer, we could cut the death rate by 75 percent. This would be 75 percent of 360,000 people who die every year of cancer. These are people whose lives could have been extended with the use of vitamin C."

Why did Dr. Cameron try vitamin C? What indications did Dr. Pauling have that vitamin C would help cancer survival?

In 1951 it was established that cancer patients have lower than average amounts of vitamin C in their blood plasma and white blood corpuscles; therefore, their weakened immune systems can't destroy cancer cells.

In 1948, epidemiologists Drs. A. C. Chope and Lester Breslow interviewed 577 older residents of San Mateo County, California. When they followed up the interviews eight years later, they found the death rate for those with the highest amounts of dietary vitamin C was less than half (40 percent) of those getting lesser amounts of vitamin C. This was true for the cancer death rate as well.

Irwin Stone reported that German physicians W. G. Deucher (1940), Von Wendt (1949), and L. Huber (1953) used 1 and 2 gram doses of vitamin C (with and without vitamin A) with good results.

Stone also reported that in 1954 Dr. W. J. McCormick found that "the degree of malignancy is determined inversely by the degree of connective tissue resistance which in turn is dependent upon the adequacy of vitamin C status."

Earlier, in 1948, Drs. Goth and Littman found that "cancers most frequently originate in organs whose vitamin C levels are below 4.5 mg percent and rarely grow in organs containing vitamin C above this concentration."

In 1966, Dr. Cameron had published his book *Hyaluronidase and Cancer* (Pergamon Press, 1966) outlining his views that strengthening the intercellular ground substance (the material that holds tissue cells together and is often called cellular cement) would prevent infiltration of cancer cells. He had noticed that cancer cells produced an enzyme, hyaluronidase, that attacked this intercellular cement and allowed the cancer to invade surrounding tissues.

In 1971 Dr. Cameron read of Dr. Pauling's comments that vitamin C increased the rate of collagen production, which strengthened the intercellular cement. This stimulated Dr. Cameron to begin cautious treatment of cancer patients with vitamin C, and the two researchers joined on some projects. One of Dr. Cameron's first observations was that vitamin C reduced the patients' pain and improved their sense of wellbeing, appetite and mental alertness. Patients who had been receiving large doses of morphine or diamorphine no longer needed the painkilling drugs.

In 1973, the Norwegian Cancer Registry's researcher, Dr. Bjelke, surveyed 30,000 people and found that the greater the intake of vitamin C, the smaller the incidence of cancer—as Drs. Chope and Breslow had found in 1948.

In 1969, Dr. Dean Burk of the National Cancer Institute found that vitamin C caused changes in cultures of cancer cells that destroyed them while being harmless to normal cells. Dr. Burk concluded, "The future of effective cancer chemotherapy will not rest on the use of host-toxic compounds now so widely employed, but upon virtually host-nontoxic compounds that are lethal to cancer cells, of which vitamin C represents an excellent prototype example."

Later that year. Dr. J. U. Schlegel of the Tulane University School of Medicine showed that bladder cancer due to smoking could be prevented by vitamin C.

In response to questions about the Cameron–Pauling report, Dr. Paul Chretien, Chief of Tumor Immunology in the Surgical branch of the National Cancer Institute, said, "It is possible they did arrest the progress of tumor growth with massive doses of vitamin C. National Cancer Institute research has shown that vitamin C given to healthy patients stimulates the body's defense system and this usually means an increased immune response."

The immune system defends the body against bacteria, viruses and other foreign invaders, as well as misformed materials in the body. It quickly recognizes, attacks and destroys all foreign bodies that can do harm.

Lymphocytes are a particular variety of white blood cell that typically make up 25 to 30 percent of all white blood cells. They can be distinguished from the typical white cells under a microscope by their lack of granules. Some lymphocytes are made in the thymus, a small gland in the neck and upper part of the chest behind the breastbone, but they are primarily made in the bone marrow. After their formation, lymphocytes are transported to the lymph nodes and spleen for lifetime storage to be used when needed. Major lymph nodes are under the arms, in the groin, behind the ears, and in the abdominal cavity and a few other places. These white blood cells are released in response to infection.

But even before the supply of lymphocytes is released in the body to fight infection, the available lymphocytes react immediately to any threat by releasing proteins called antibodies. After antibodies attack the invader, larger cells called macrophages are summoned to "chew up" the invader. Both antibodies and lymphocytes are released in response to the presence of cancerous cells.

Dr. Chretien's comment on the immune system referred to

research he conducted with his NCI colleague Dr. T. F. Tehniger and Dr. Robert Yonemoto, Director of Surgical Laboratories at the City of Hope National Medical Center in Duarte, California. The researchers were looking for a solution to a perplexing problem of cancer surgery. Immediately after the surgical removal of malignant tumors, the immune system is very weak. Often cancer cells spill into the bloodstream during surgery, and when the immune response is weak the spilled cancer cells spread secondary cancers—metastases—throughout the body.

The group published a study in 1976 showing that 5 grams of vitamin C daily increased the production of lymphocytes (white blood corpuscles without granules) when the body was threatened by a foreign substance, and that 10 grams daily produced an even greater effect. Cancer patients have a poor capacity for making new lymphocytes, yet their ability to survive relates strongly to their lymphocyte production.

The study subjects were healthy volunteers, and the researchers are now studying cancer patients to see if the same results can be observed.

All studies discussed so far have been with people. Preliminary cancer research is normally carried out with laboratory animals such as rats and mice, but there is a great difference with respect to vitamin C between humans and most animals. Most animals make their own vitamin C or at least make most of what they need. Man, primates, guinea pigs and a few other animals cannot produce vitamin C because of the lack of a required enzyme, believed to be caused by a genetic abnormality developed during evolution.

The guinea pig is a suitable experimental animal for vitamin C research, but not much is known about cancer in guinea pigs, although Dr. George Feigen, professor of physiology at Stanford University, in studying the effects of vitamin C on their immune systems, has observed a large increase in the production of one of the components of the immune response.

Previously, researchers at the Bowman Gray School of Medicine in Winston-Salem, North Carolina reported that vitamin C activated the immune response. At the June 1971 meeting of the American Society of Biological Chemists in San Francisco, Drs. Lawrence R. DeChatelet, Charles E. McCall and M. Robert Cooper reported that adding vitamin C to test-tube mixtures of white corpuscles and bacteria stimulated increased activity of the white blood corpuscles. Without the added vitamin C, the white blood corpuscles can engulf the bacteria, but they cannot break them down.

All these reports illustrate the fact that vitamin C boosts immunity, which is the body's most important line of defense against cancer.

In 1983, Dr. Bernard Kennes of the Université Libre de Bruxelles in Belgium, reported that the immune system of elderly persons could be significantly enhanced with 500 milligrams of vitamin C daily. In *Gerontology* (29:305-310, 1983) he concludes, "vitamin C should be considered as a possible successful, nontoxic and inexpensive substance that improves the immune competence of the aging."

ANTIOXIDANT COMBINATIONS ARE BETTER

Combinations of antioxidants provide better protection than might be expected when considering each antioxidant individually; the effect is synergistic, an example of the whole being greater than the sum of its parts. In my experiments I found that combinations of vitamins A, C and E plus the trace mineral selenium were more effective than larger amounts of the individual antioxidant nutrients. This observation was the basis of several world-wide patents that I applied for in the early 1970s. This research and much more about the role of antioxidants against cancer, along with the evidence, is described in my book *Cancer and Its Nutritional Therapies* (Keats Publishing, 1978, 1983).

The importance of the antioxidant nutrients has recently been recognized by the National Cancer Institute and the American Cancer Society. Studies are now under way to explore further the roles of selenium and beta-carotene in countering cancer in humans.

WHAT IS AGING?

The American Medical Association's Committee on Aging has studied the problem of human aging for more than a decade. The committee has so far not found one physical or mental condition that can be directly attributed simply to the passage of time. Some of the alleged diseases of aging—such as high blood pressure and arthritis—are prevalent in the very young as well as the very old. What exactly *is* aging, then, and what are its causes?

Aging can be described as the process that reduces the number of healthy cells in the body. Although we have noted the increase of some enzymes in the body and the decrease of others, the most striking factor in the aging process is the body's loss of reserve due to the decreasing amount of cells in each organ. For example, fasting blood glucose levels remain fairly constant throughout life, but the glucose tolerance measurement, which measures the reserve capacity of this system to respond to the stress of the glucose load, shows a loss of response with aging. The same holds true concerning the recovery mechanisms of other parameters.

Cellular aging actually begins before birth and is the one factor underlying the aging process of the entire body. The stability of the living system becomes progressively impaired by chemical reactions, not the passage of time.

If we can control the rate of these deleterious reactions, then we can control the advance of physiological aging.

Free-radical reactions, discussed earlier, result in the loss of active cells. The cumulative effect of billions of cellular free-radical reactions is to add to the body's loss of reserve. Again, that is what the aging process is—the loss of reserve function.

Not only are antioxidant nutrients protective against cancer, they can slow the aging process or at least slow its acceleration. This is not to suggest that antioxidants will rejuvenate you. It means that they will help protect you against the damage that adds signs of aging to your body.

My experiments have shown that certain combinations of antioxidant nutrients can extend the average lifespan of laboratory animals by 20 to 30 percent, and the maximum lifespan by 5 to 10 percent. In experiments in which laboratory conditions were designed to accelerate the aging process, the antioxidants increased the lifespans of the animals by as much as 175 percent.

Other researchers such as Dr. Denham Harman of the University of Nebraska School of Medicine, England's Dr. Alex Comfort and Dr. Al Tappel of the University of California at Davis have found that individual antioxidant nutrients produce significant lifespan increases, though less than that of the synergistic combinations.

Antioxidant nutrients help prevent heart disease by protecting the arteries against the damage that leads to the cholesterol deposits called plaque, but the risk of heart attacks is more significantly decreased by the nutrients' ability to keep fatal blood clots from forming in the coronary arteries.

Let's consider both these roles of the antioxidant nutrients. Dr. Earl Benditt of the University of Washington discovered that the cholesterol-containing plaque in the lining of arteries actually begins as a mutated muscle cell in the middle layer of the artery.

In my view, the mutation described by Dr. Benditt is caused by free radicals. My research centers on free radicals and their involvement in accelerating aging and initiating cancer and heart disease. Dr. Benditt's observations explain the link between free-radical production and heart disease found in experiments.

The overall process in plaque formation then is as follows: The initial plaque formed is due to a mutation of a cell in the artery wall. Certain chemicals in the bloodstream, including pollutants, smoke components, and free radicals cause a normal smooth muscle cell in the arterial wall to go haywire (mutate).

The cell that mutated because of the reactive chemicals reproduces itself (proliferates) precisely. All derived cells are exact replicas (monoclonal) and form a growth differing from normal artery tissue. This growth, the first step in plaque formation, has been missed by other researchers.

The plaque now develops in stages. In stage one, the proliferating smooth muscle cells spread through the artery wall, causing the production of extracellular substances including collagen (a structural protein) and glycosaminoglycans (carbohydrates).

Monoclonal proliferation continues at a fast rate until cell crowding results. At this stage, cholesterol is manufactured by the crowded cell as a result of cellular injury from the overcrowding of monoclonal cells. This second stage produces the uncomplicated plaque that for a century has been wrongly considered characteristic of the first stage.

The third stage is a complication of the second stage; in it, the fibrous mass protrudes through the arterial wall where it comes into contact with the flowing blood; calcium and additional cholesterol from the bloodstream can now add to the fibrous plaque. This third stage is independent of blood cholesterol level, but may be related to the concentration of low-density lipoprotein (LDL) in the blood.

In 1974, Swedish researcher Dr. K. Korsan-Bengsten, of the medical department of the Sahlgrens Hospital in Göteborg, reported that vitamin E returns abnormal platelets to normal.

Brown University researchers Drs. Manfred Steiner and John Anastasi reported in the *Journal of Clinical Investigation* (March 1976) that platelet adhesion was reduced as the dosage of tocopherol was increased to a level of 1,800 International Units (IU). In the men and women tested, platelet adhesion was lowered by as much as 50 percent.

The mechanism by which vitamin E normalizes blood platelets to reduce their stickiness involves the production of prostaglandin X. Prostaglandins are hormone-like compounds that control many body functions (sometimes banefully, as with arthritis). Prostaglandin X is manufactured in the artery linings and converts damaged platelets back to normal. Vitamin E increases prostaglandin X production, while the peroxidized polyunsaturated fats inhibit it (Moncade et al., *Lancet*, 1977).

The action of vitamin E in keeping blood free-flowing so that coronaries are reduced explains why vitamin E lowers the incidence of heart disease in long-term users. In *Supernutrition for Healthy Hearts* (1977) I report the results of my study of 17,894 people showing that the amount of heart disease in any age group decreased proportionally with the length of time the participants took vitamin E.

Two groups in the survey well illustrate this point. One group consisted of those who had taken 400 IU or more of vitamin E daily for ten years or more. The study included 2,508 such people between the ages of 50 and 98. Based on Department of Health, Education and Welfare figures (HRS 74-1222, 1976), normally 836 of the 2,508 would be expected to have heart disease. Instead there were only four. This is less than one percent of the expected number.

A second group of 1,038 had taken 1,200 IU or more of vitamin E daily for four years or more. In this group (differing slightly from the first in age-group composition), normally there would be 323 suffering from heart disease rather than the seven actually found.

Vitamin E has been found to greatly increase the beneficial blood component high-density lipoprotein (HDL). We owe this most important discovery to the alertness of Dr. W. J. Hermann of Memorial City General Hospital in Houston.

Dr. Hermann found that his HDL ratio increased from 9

percent to 40 percent after taking 600 IU of vitamin E for one month. Realizing the importance of this observation, he recruited ten volunteers for a clinical trial to see if the incredible improvement was a general response to vitamin E.

Five of the volunteers had normal HDL levels prior to taking vitamin E and five had low HDL levels. Thirty days of taking 600 IU of vitamin E brought about significant improvement in HDL levels in both groups. Those having normal HDL levels averaged a 50 percent improvement, while those with low HDL levels averaged a whopping 200 percent increase.

The results were published by Dr. Hermann and his colleagues, Drs. K. Ward and J. Faucett, in the *American Journal of Clinical Pathology* in late 1979.

Drs. Evan and Wilfrid Shute taught for thirty years that vitamin E was helpful to those with heart disease because it was anti-clotting, improved oxygen utilization, controlled the patch-scar that replaces damaged heart tissue, and improved capillary permeability. Some physicians found similar results in their practices; others did not. Perhaps those that did not have success with vitamin E did not use it long enough for the platelet normalization effect to occur. The new findings about prostaglandin X and platelets should end the confusion.

However, pounds of vitamin E will not protect you if you are deficient in other nutrients or fail to follow the ideal lifestyle of moderation. The antioxidant mineral selenium is required as a partner for vitamin E. Reasonable amounts of vitamin E for those seeking protection are 400 IU daily and up to 800 IU daily for control. Reasonable recommendations for selenium are 50 micrograms daily for protection and 100 mcg daily for control. These are only general recommendations. Because of individual variations in diet, lifestyle and genetic background, the optimum level will differ for each individual. Several nutrients help control blood pressure. Selenium and vitamin E are especially important. A selenium deficiency causes a harmful compound to build up in the blood that increases blood pressure. Selenium is involved in the production of several prostaglandins which regulate blood pressure. When there is a selenium deficiency, a critical enzyme that contains selenium is not produced, and as a result an intermediate compound in the production of prostaglandin accumulates. When this intermediate compound is in excess, blood pressure is increased.

The pain, swelling and inflammation of arthritis are also caused by free radicals. Human studies in Great Britain have found that approximately 80 percent of arthritis sufferers found significant relief from pain and reduced swelling and inflammation by taking the combination of antioxidant nutrients, vitamins A, C and E, plus the trace mineral selenium. This study was undertaken when the head of a British arthritis group noticed that his arthritis symptoms disappeared after he had been taking the antioxidants for a time for another reason. The placebo effect can be discounted because the person was not taking the antioxidant nutrients in an effort to control his arthritis.

One hundred other members of the British Arthritic Association were asked to try the antioxidant nutrients, and after initial success, a larger study involving 418 members was undertaken.

In Israel, a double-blind crossover study in which 600 milligrams of vitamin E or placebo were given for ten days to osteoarthritis patients found that more than 50 percent of the patients had significant relief from pain during the vitamin E period compared to only 4 percent during the placebo period.

At the May 1980 meeting of selenium researchers, Norwegian scientists reported the beneficial results of selenium in arthritis patients. The researchers found that the rheumatoid arthritis patients had lower-than-normal levels of selenium in their blood. Supplementation with selenium and vitamin E brought about significant reduction in symptoms.

Another physician at this conference, Dr. E. Crary of Smyrna, Georgia, had also treated patients having traumatic arthritis with selenium and the vitamins A, C and E, successfully relieving the pain in their traumatized joints.

These favorable results could have been predicted from the knowledge that the free-radical scavenger superoxide dismutase has been proven highly successful against arthritis. In tissues, free radicals generate superoxide radicals and lipoperoxides that promote the release of the deleterious prostaglandins that cause pain, inflammation and swelling. Selenium (in the enzyme glutathione peroxidase) protects against this damage, as do other antioxidants. In addition, vitamin E directly decreases the output of the deleterious postaglandins.

The anti-inflammatory action of selenium has been widely accepted in animal treatment. Injectable and oral veterinary formulations of vitamin E and selenium have been used for years. Several such preparations are FDA-approved for symptomatic relief of arthritic inflammation in dogs. Topical vitamin E has been shown to have anti-inflammatory action in rats and rabbits.

CATARACTS

Recent research has linked antioxidant deficiencies to cataract development. The antioxidants normally protect the sensitive proteins in the eye lens. When there isn't sufficient antioxidant protection, the proteins can oxidize in the lens, causing it to cloud and scatter light.

Antioxidant levels in a cataracted lens are a fraction of those in a healthy lens. Several researchers have found that they can slow or halt the growth of cataracts by having their patients take supplements of the antioxidant nutrients, thus normalizing the antioxidant levels of the lens.

Dr. Alex Duarte of the Cataract Control Center in Huntington Beach, California, has written a book describing the role of free radicals in the production of cataracts and how the antioxidant nutrients are protective. His book *Cataract Breakthrough* (International Institute of Natural Health Sciences, Inc. P.O. Box 5550, Huntington Beach, California) also describes the treatment for the cure of cataracts.

ALLERGIES

Chemical hypersensitivities are often caused by free-radical reactions. Some seemingly inert chemicals can be converted into potent free-radical generators by the actions of body enzymes as they metabolize the foreign chemicals in an attempt to remove them from the body. Many people who are allergic (sensitive) to various chemicals have found that their allergies disappeared soon after taking antioxidant nutrients for some other reason such as protection against cancer or heart disease.

Dr. Stephen A. Levine of the Allergy Research Group in Pleasant Hill, California is one such individual. He suffered considerably until he started taking antioxidants in 1980. Now he has studied the mechanisms fully and has published his clinical observations in the *Journal of Orthomolecular Psychiatry* and the *Allergy Research Review.*

HOW MUCH?

The amount of each antioxidant required for protection against the various free-radical pathologies varies from individual to individual and with the total nutrition and lifestyle of the individual. The first consideration is whether a deficiency does exist. The following table lists the Recommended Dietary Allowance (to determine deficiency) and a safe and effective range to consider for therapeutic supplementation.

Nutrient Range	RDA	Supplementation
Vitamin A	5,000 IU (RE)	5,000-25,000 IU
Beta-carotene	(included in the above for vitamin A)	10,000-20,000 IU
Vitamin C	60 mg.	500-2,000 mg
Vitamin E	15 IU	50-600 IU
Selenium	50-200 mcg	100-200 mcg

BIBLIOGRAPHY

Hailey, Herbert. *E, the Essential Vitamin.* New York: Bantam Books, 1983.

Cameron, Ewan and Linus Pauling. *Cancer and Vitamin C.* New York: Warner Books, 1981.

Hoffer, Abram and Morton Walker. *Orthomolecular Nutrition.* New Canaan, Conn.: Keats Publishing, 1978.

Kugler, Hans. *Seven Keys to a Longer Life.* Briarcliff Manor, N.Y.: Stein & Day, 1978.

Passwater, Richard A. *Cancer and Its Nutritional Therapies.* New Canaan, Conn.: Keats Publishing, 1983.

―――. *EPA—Marine Lipids.* New Canaan, Conn.: Keats Publishing, 1982.

―――. *Selenium as Food and Medicine.* New Canaan, Conn.: Keats Publishing, 1980.

―――. *Supernutrition for Healthy Hearts.* New York: Dial Press, 1977.

Pryor, W. *Free Radicals.* New York: McGraw-Hill Publishing Co., 1966.

Spallholz, Martin and Ganther, eds. *Selenium in Biology and Medicine.* Westport, Conn.: AVI Press, 1981.